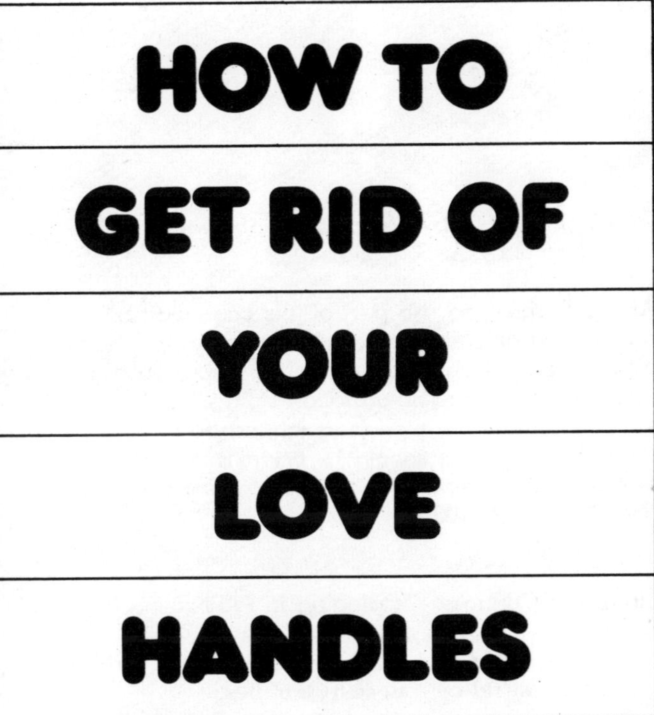

Betty Ann Hightower

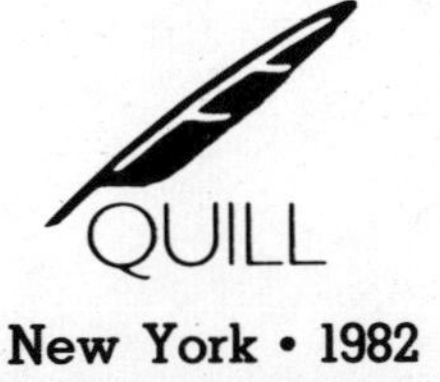

New York • 1982

Photographs by A. S. Collins

Library of Congress Cataloging in Publication Data

Hightower, Betty Ann.
How to get rid of your love handles.

1. Reducing exercises. 2. Exercises for women.
3. Hip joint. I. Title.
[RA781.6.H53 1982] 646.7'5 82-9035
ISBN 0-688-01357-0 (pbk.) AACR2

Printed in the United States of America

5 6 7 8 9 10

Book Design by Liney Li

LOVE HANDLES

Mikhail Baryshnikov and Bjorn Borg do not have love handles. Neither do other ballet and tennis stars, gymnasts, broad jumpers, pole-vaulters, and slalom skiers. If you have ever watched a ballet, a professional tennis match, or a gymnastic or jumping competition, you have seen the results of years of constant work at keeping fit. Each of these activities requires not only general fitness and flexibility, but also a great deal of bending and flexing of the muscles at the sides of the waist. Participation in general exercise programs and sports such as golf, swimming, baseball, and cross-country skiing is no guarantee that love handles will disappear. These unsightly bulges at the sides of your waist won't go away unless you do exercises and activities that really develop the muscles in that area.

How can you tell if you have love handles? The pinch test and the mirror test are two easy ways to answer the question. You have love handles if you can pinch more than an inch of flesh at the sides of your waist, in the area between your rib cage and your hipbones. Sagging folds at the sides of your waist are the surest sign, but don't despair if you see them in the mirror. You can get rid of your love handles if you are willing to spend a few minutes a day doing exercises specifically aimed at making them vanish.

Before beginning a program to get rid of your love handles, you should understand the causes of the problem. The complex arrangement of lateral muscles in your midsection enables you to bend and flex your torso. Nature has provided you with an efficient structural support system, a natural girdle composed of overlapping and crisscrossing muscle fibers. The muscles involved in the problem of love handles are the external and interal oblique muscles and the transversus abdominis muscle, which can be seen in the illustrations. The long muscle in the front of the abdomen, the rectus abdominis, is also shown because it is inserted into the transversus abdominis, and because it controls the tilt of the pelvis.

The external, or descending, oblique muscle is the outermost of the three. It is attached on each side of the body to the lower eight ribs and descends inward at an angle. The lower fibers of the muscle are attached to the crest of the ilium, which is part of the hipbone. The upper and middle fibers of the external obliques from both sides of the body meet at the midline, where they are attached not to a bone, but to a ribbonlike tendon.

Beneath the external oblique muscle is the internal oblique, whose fibers are somewhat thinner than those of the external oblique and which lies at a diagonal to it. If you look at the illustrations of the external and internal obliques and picture the former placed over the latter, you will see that they crisscross.

The innermost lateral muscle, the transversus abdominis, is named for the direction of its fibers; they traverse—that is, cross—the waist and meet in the back. This muscle is attached in part to the ilium and in part to the rib cartilage and ligaments of the lower spine.

Unlike muscles in other parts of the body, not all of these muscles have a bone as their second attachment. This

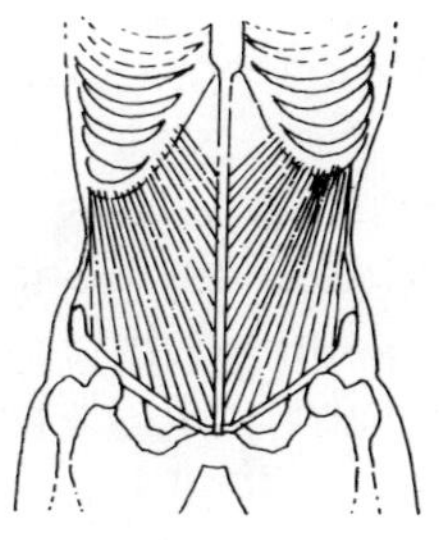
External oblique

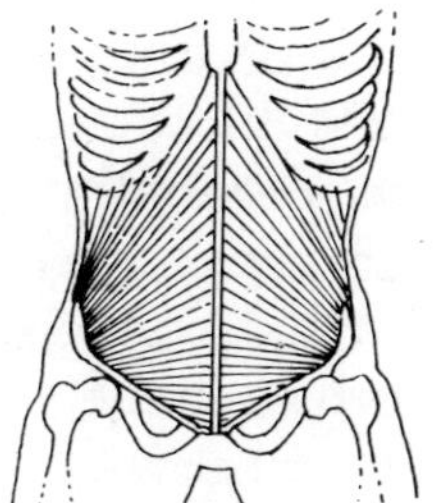
Internal oblique

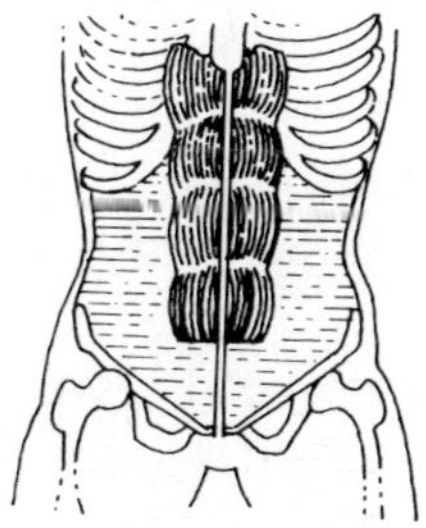
Rectus abdominis

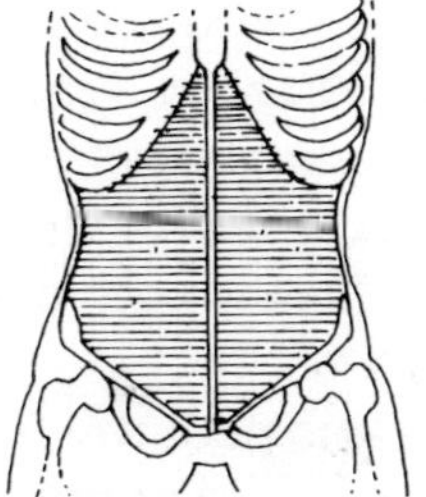
Transversus abdominis

arrangement allows you to flex your torso freely. (Compare this with your finger muscles, which securely and tightly connect bone to bone. You probably can easily bend your fingers, but you cannot comfortably twist them like your torso.) Parts of these long lateral muscles lie along the sides of your body, and when they slacken and bulge due to lack of exercise, love handles are the result. Taut and strong lateral muscles, on the other hand, mean no love handles.

How often do you twist, bend, stretch, and exercise

your torso during your workday? Unless you participate in sports that exercise these muscles, you probably engage in very few activities that can keep love handles from developing. It almost seems as if the features of modern life conspire against our keeping fit and trim. Our normal daily routines don't require enough physical exertion, and we must compensate for that lack. To get rid of love handles, it is necessary to do exercises designed to flex, stretch, and tighten the lateral muscles of the waist. That is what the exercise program in this book is designed to do.

One important factor contributing to the problem of love handles is excessive fat. If many people at their ideal weight have love handles—and they do—you can easily imagine what cushions of excess fat over and around slack muscles can do to complicate the problem. Therefore, if you are overweight, it is very important to diet in addition to exercising.

Another factor that may exaggerate your love-handle problem is posture. Take a look at yourself in a full-length mirror to check how you normally stand. Do you slouch? Do your shoulders droop? Do you tend to hang your head? Does your abdomen stick out? Do you let your midsection collapse when you sit?

If you answered yes to any of these questions, your posture needs improvement. Try to stand straight while also holding your head up. Imagine a straight line from the back of your head to your heels. Tuck in your abdomen and square your shoulders. You will notice that your love handles become less prominent. Standing straight will help to keep your waist trim.

HOW TO USE THIS EXERCISE PROGRAM

It is advisable to consult a physician before undertaking any exercise program if you have a serious back condition or other medical problems that restrict physical activity in any way.

Once you have decided to begin the program, you have taken a big step. At this point, it is important to establish a regular time and comfortable place for exercise. While it is possible to do many of these exercises in various rooms of your home or even in your office, you may become careless about the exercises if you think of them merely as casual, spare-time activities. Do extra exercises whenever and wherever you can, but be sure to set up a regular schedule and stick to it. It doesn't matter if you miss an occasional day as long as you resume the routine the following day. It is the *routine* that is important. If you set aside 15 to 20 minutes a day, your efforts will pay off!

Wear comfortable, loose-fitting clothing, underwear, leotards, or shorts when you exercise. Some of the exercises can be done in any type of apparel, but most of them require clothing that does not restrict movement. Since a number of the exercises are to be done on the floor, use a mat if you don't have a carpet.

Don't begin an exercise until you are completely familiar with its movements. Carefully read the instructions and examine the demonstration photographs. Remember, muscles will not get stronger without stress. As you do an exercise, you should be able to feel your muscles flexing or stretching and contracting, but not to the point of strain or, worse, pain. Do the exercises slowly and smoothly to avoid the discomfort and strain that are sometimes caused by rushed and jerky movements. Above all, don't force a movement. Some bodies are naturally more flexible than others, and straining oneself can be counterproductive. If a particular movement causes you pain, your body is sending you a message—"Stop, something's wrong!" Do not do any exercise that is painful to you. If you do strain yourself slightly, moist heat, massage, and reduction in the number of exercises or repetitions will help to relieve some of the soreness you may experience.

Remember that it will take time to achieve results and that different body types will shape up at different rates. Be sensible and patient. You can't rush the process.

THE PROGRAM

This systematic approach to eliminating your love handles begins with some useful Warm-ups and then explains exercises on several levels of difficulty. Each level leads to the next, but not everyone must start with Level 1. A self-evaluation of your general fitness, flexibility, and life-style will help you determine the appropriate starting level for you. No one who isn't in the very best physical condition should start with Level 3. If you are fairly active—that is, if you play tennis, soccer, handball, or racquetball regularly or if your job requires strenuous physical activity—you can begin at Level 2. Begin at Level 1 if you have a desk job or if you consider yourself unathletic. Once you have tried some of the activities from Level 1, you may decide that you are fitter than you at first thought. But it is a good idea to start safely at Level 1.

Set aside at least ten minutes a day for the exercises. During each session do at least five exercises following the Warm-ups. When you are familiar with the exercises, try the Warm-ups and each Level 1 exercise five times. If you find the five repetitions *very* easy, make sure that you are doing the exercises correctly before you increase the number of repetitions or attempt new exercises. Check yourself in a mirror. Is your back straight when it should be? Are you swaying your pelvis or tilting forward when you shouldn't? Add three to five repetitions if you did the exercises correctly and found them very easy. The average beginner should not take on too many repetitions or additional exercises. It even may be necessary to start more slowly than suggested above.

Some exercises may come easily; others will seem impossible at first; a few may never be within your physical ability. For example, you may have an easy time with the Level 1 Twist, Slide, Hoop, and Lift, but the Sidesaddle may seem extremely hard and the Level 3 one-arm Triangle impossible. When you can do ten repetitions of at least four exercises from Level 1, you can begin Level 2.

At Levels 2 and 3 you may wish to follow up the Warm-ups with a few exercises from previous levels, but with additional repetitions. Introduce a new exercise with no more than five repetitions unless you find it very easy. At the end of your exercise session, stretch your arms overhead and bend to the left and right several times. Relax your arms at your sides and do the Roundabout slowly to cool down.

In the first two weeks of the program, do more exercises with fewer repetitions (five to eight exercises plus Warm-ups, with five to ten repetitions). As your midsection gets firmer, increase the number of repetitions and do fewer exercises.

It is important to incorporate some of these exercises into your general exercise program after you have achieved the goal of getting rid of your love handles. Do any 5 of the exercises from Levels 1, 2, and 3 that you found moderately difficult about 15 times each, which should take roughly 6 minutes altogether. You can alternate exercises, but to keep your love handles from returning, continue to work out every other day.

EXERCISE INSTRUCTIONS: NOTES AND DEFINITIONS

Torso: The trunk of the body, to which the head and limbs are attached.

Pelvis: The lower portion of the torso, bounded at the sides and in front by the ilium and in back by the fused vertebrae, or sacrum, in the lower back.

It is important to understand why the position of the pelvis must be stable to obtain good results from some of these exercises. Turn to the Level 1 Twist and try the exercise with your hands on your hipbones. First do the exercise this way: keep your pelvis as still and straight as you can. Then do it a second time, letting your pelvis sway or tilt back. The stable position of the pelvis provides much greater pull on the muscles; the tilting or swaying is counterproductive. The instructions for each exercise will tell you to "keep your pelvis stable" where applicable.

Reverse: Do the exercise on the opposite side. If the instructions specify the right side and left arm, then the reverse is the left side and right arm.

Repeat: All of the instructions give the minimum number of exercise repetitions for that level. This number may be adjusted to your own physical performance abilities.

WARM~UPS

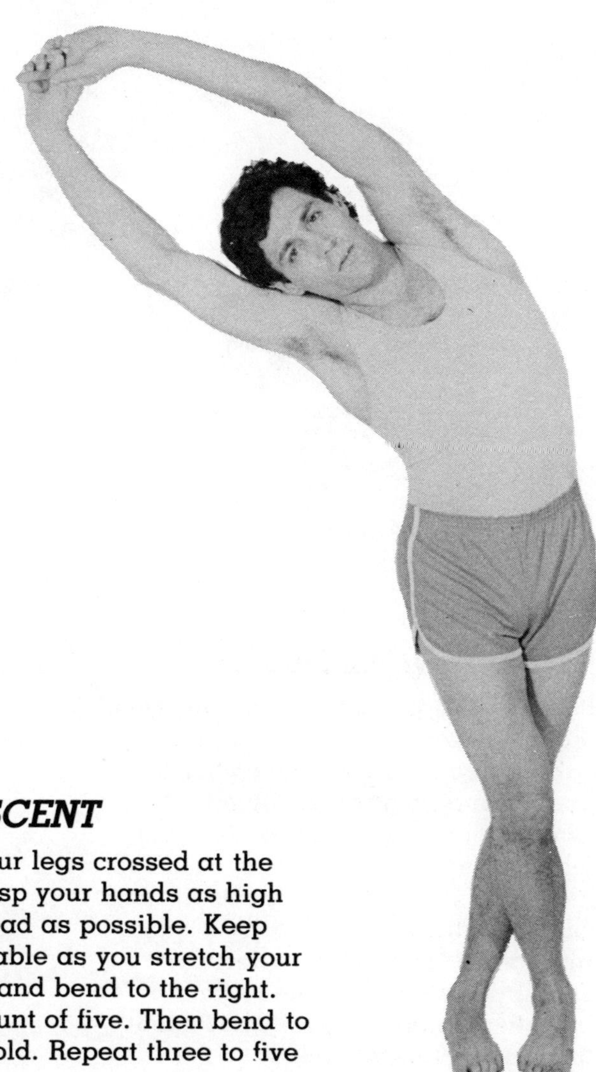

THE CRESCENT

Stand with your legs crossed at the knees and clasp your hands as high above your head as possible. Keep your pelvis stable as you stretch your torso upward and bend to the right. Hold to the count of five. Then bend to the left and hold. Repeat three to five times.

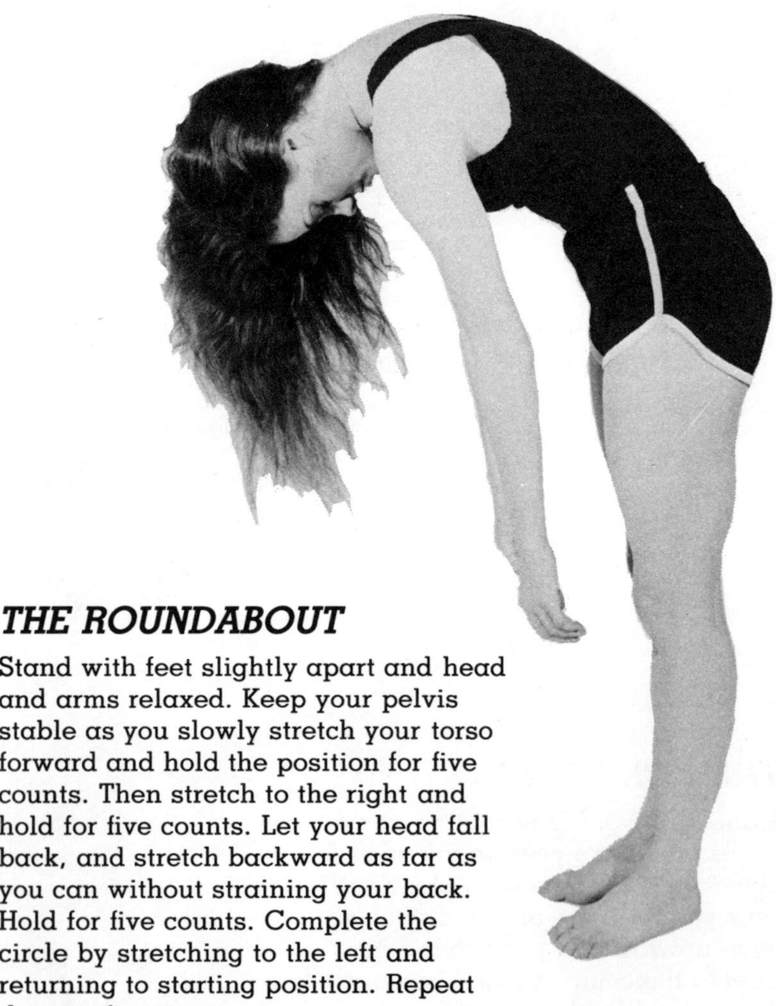

THE ROUNDABOUT

Stand with feet slightly apart and head and arms relaxed. Keep your pelvis stable as you slowly stretch your torso forward and hold the position for five counts. Then stretch to the right and hold for five counts. Let your head fall back, and stretch backward as far as you can without straining your back. Hold for five counts. Complete the circle by stretching to the left and returning to starting position. Repeat three to five times.

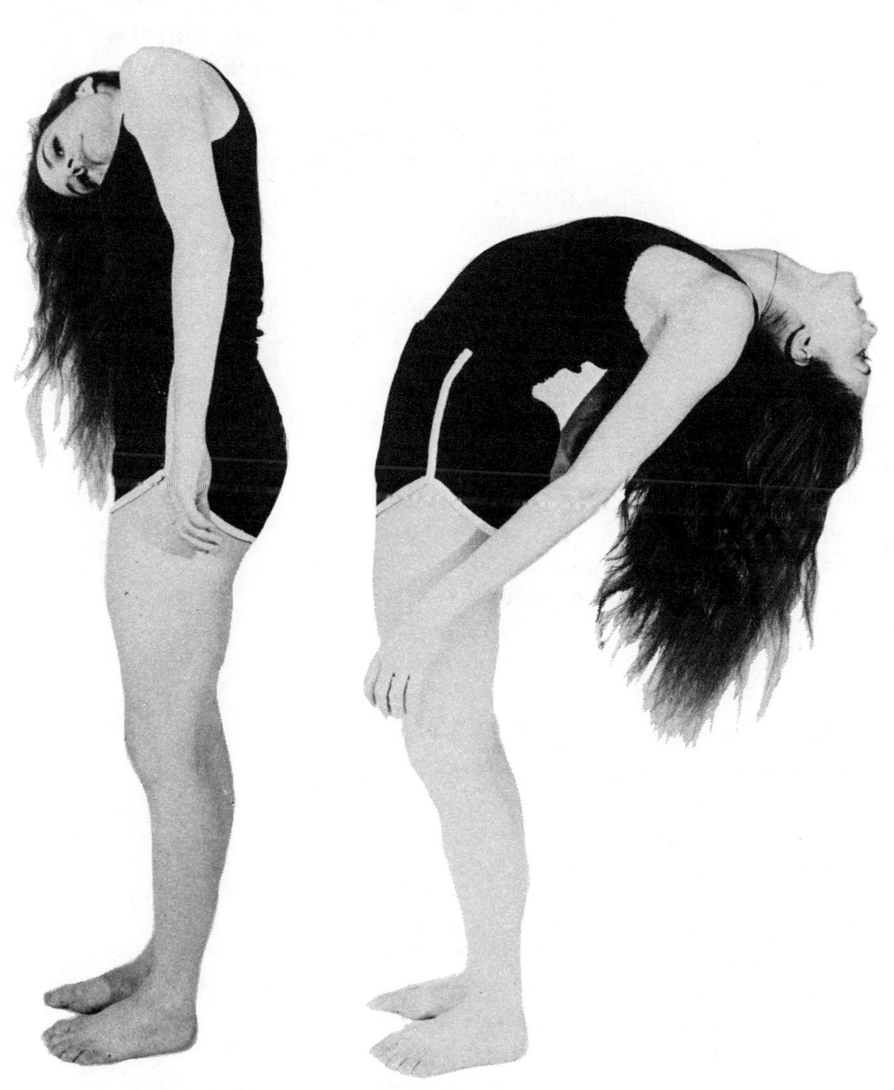

THE ROCKER

Bend your right knee and clasp your hands around it at the shin. Pull the knee as close as you can to the left side of your chest. Hold the position for five counts. Repeat three to five times. Reverse hand and leg positions and repeat.

THE GRIP

Stand with your weight on your right leg, steadying yourself with your right hand on a wall, table, or sturdy chair. Bend your left knee and grasp your left foot with your left hand. Then raise the leg back as far as you can without losing your balance. Move your body forward at the hip as you pull your leg higher and higher. Repeat three to five times. Reverse and repeat.

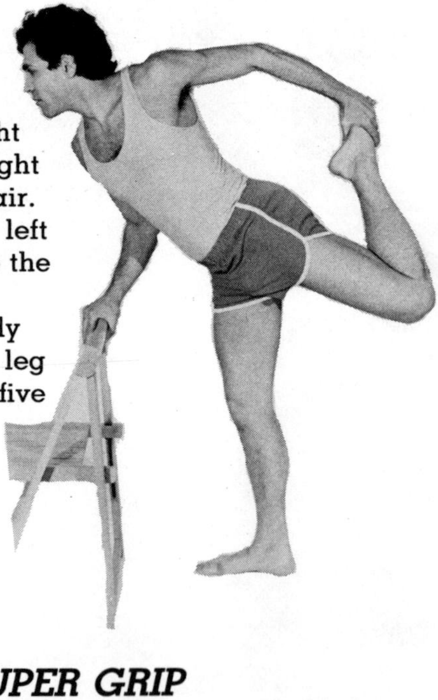

THE SUPER GRIP

This exercise is a crisscross version of the Grip. Stand with your weight on your right leg, using your left hand to steady yourself. Bring your left leg back but grasp your left foot with your *right* hand. Pull your leg as high as you can. Repeat three to five times. Reverse and repeat.

LEVEL 1

THE TWIST

Kneel with knees apart and arms outstretched to the sides. Keep your pelvis stable. Twist your torso to the left as far as possible, hold for three counts, and return to center position. Then twist to the right and hold. Repeat five times. Try the exercise with hands on hips to check your pelvis position.

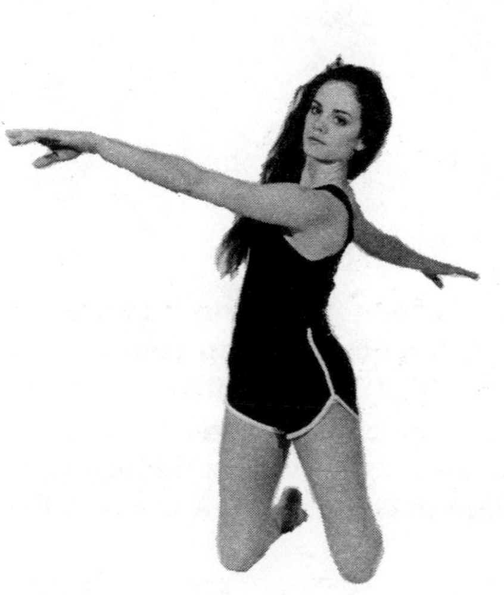

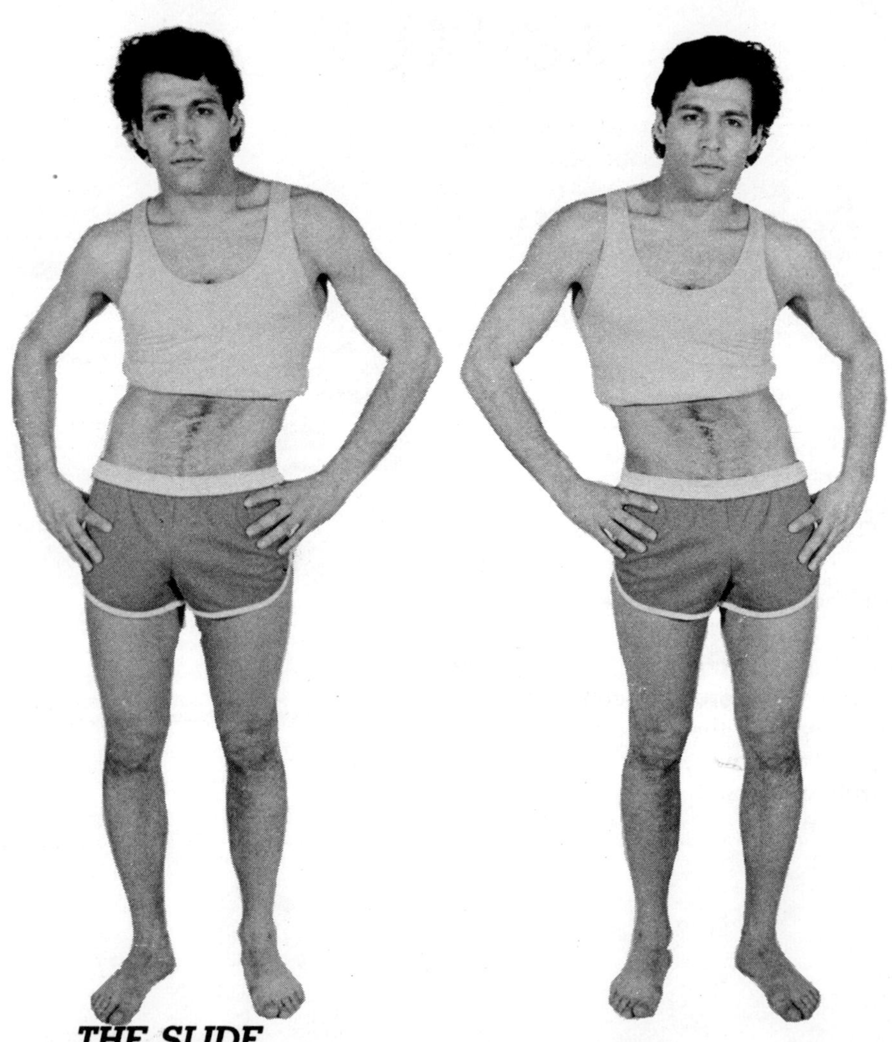

THE SLIDE

Stand with feet apart and hands on hips. Tuck in your stomach by contracting your stomach muscles. Shift your pelvis to the right *without moving your torso,* and hold to the count of five. You will feel the pull in your muscles as you do this. Return to center position and perform the exercise on the left. Repeat five times.

THE HOOP

Stand with feet wide apart and hands on hips. Lean to the left as far as you can. Moving your pelvis, circle to the front, right, back, and left as if you were twirling a hoop about your body. Repeat five times. Circle in the opposite direction five times.

THE LIFT

Lie on the floor on your left side with head resting on your extended left arm. Slowly raise your right leg as high as you can and then lower it. Repeat five times. Reverse and repeat.

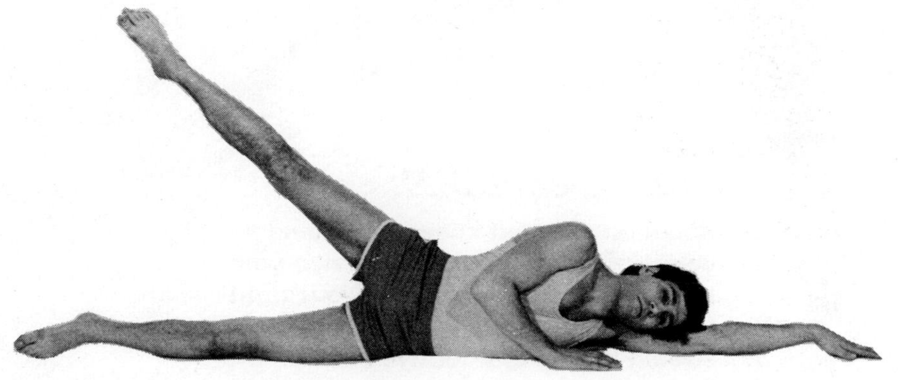

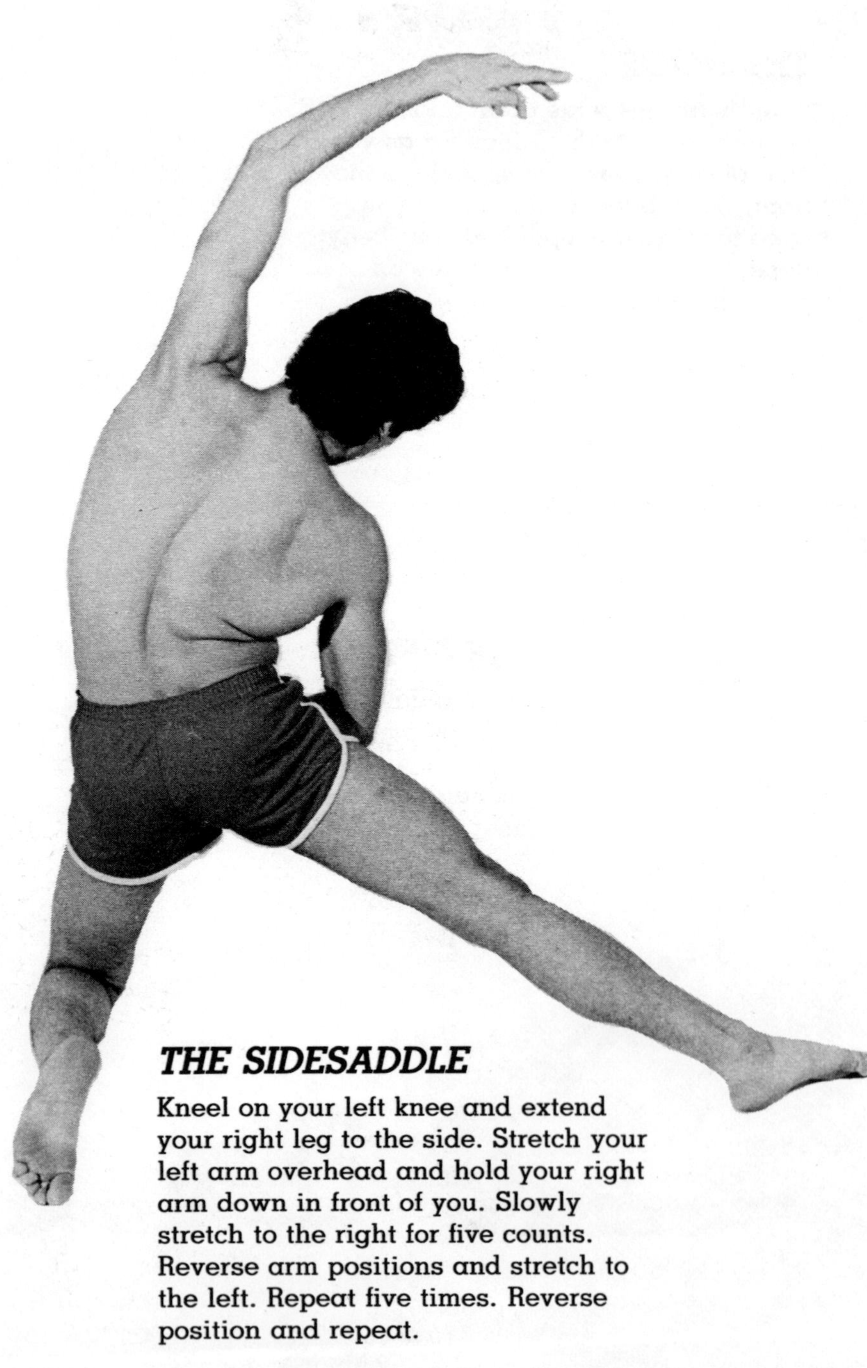

THE SIDESADDLE

Kneel on your left knee and extend your right leg to the side. Stretch your left arm overhead and hold your right arm down in front of you. Slowly stretch to the right for five counts. Reverse arm positions and stretch to the left. Repeat five times. Reverse position and repeat.

LEVEL 2

THE REARVIEW REACH

Kneel on both knees and extend both arms in front of you. Twist to the right as far as you can and reach back as if picking up some imaginary object. Hold the position for five counts. Then twist to the left, reach back, and hold. Repeat five times.

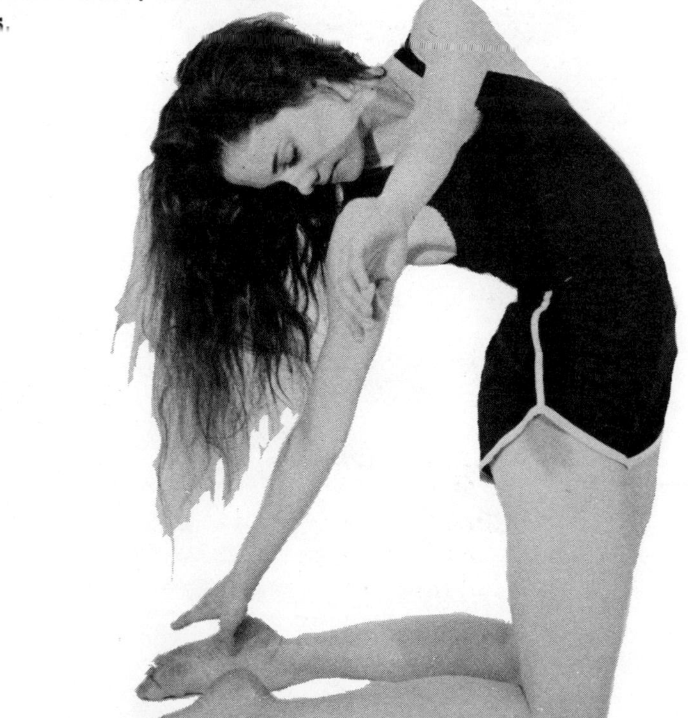

THE CROSSOVER

Lie on your back with arms outstretched. Raise your right leg toward the ceiling. Then cross your right leg over your left and touch the floor with your right leg. Repeat five times. Reverse and repeat.

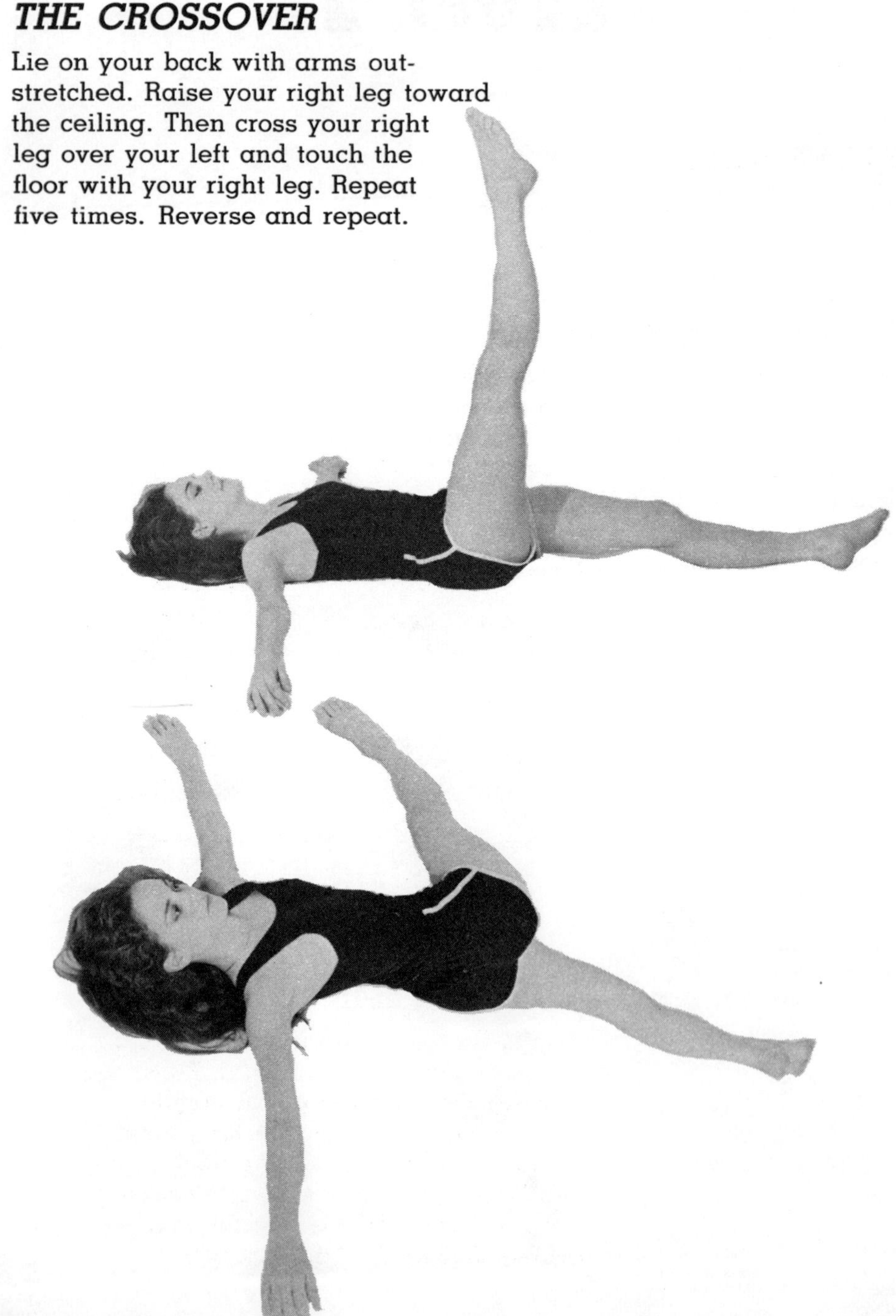

THE MERMAID

Lie on your right side with head resting on your extended right arm. Keeping your legs together, slowly raise them a few inches off the floor. Hold for five counts. Repeat five times. Reverse and repeat.

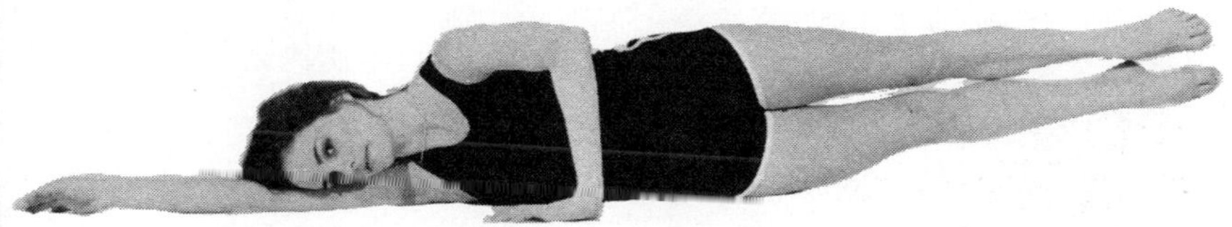

THE OVER EASY

Stand with feet comfortably apart and arms extended in front of you. Twist your torso to the right as far as you can without moving your pelvis. Bend forward and try to touch the floor with both hands, but do not force the movement. Return to center position and reverse. Repeat five times.

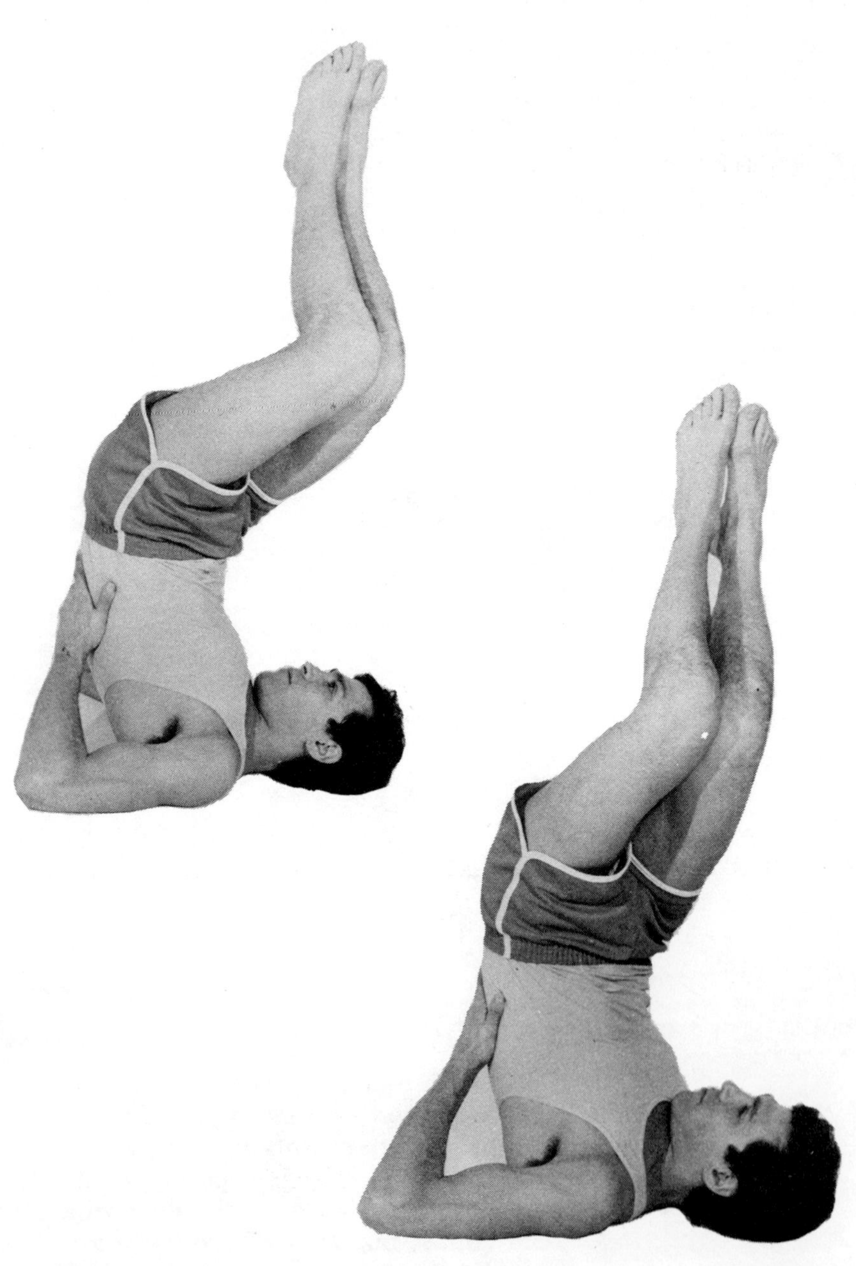

THE TAILSPIN

Lie on your back and bend your knees. Raise your torso off the floor into a shoulder stand. Support your torso at the waist with your hands, but keep your elbows on the floor. Twist your pelvis to the right and extend your legs into the air. Then bend your knees, twist to the left, and extend. Repeat five times.

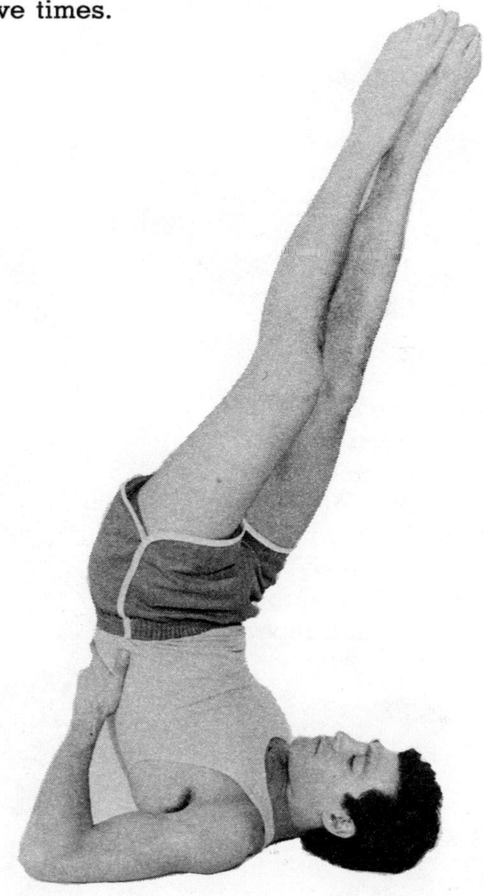

LEVEL 3

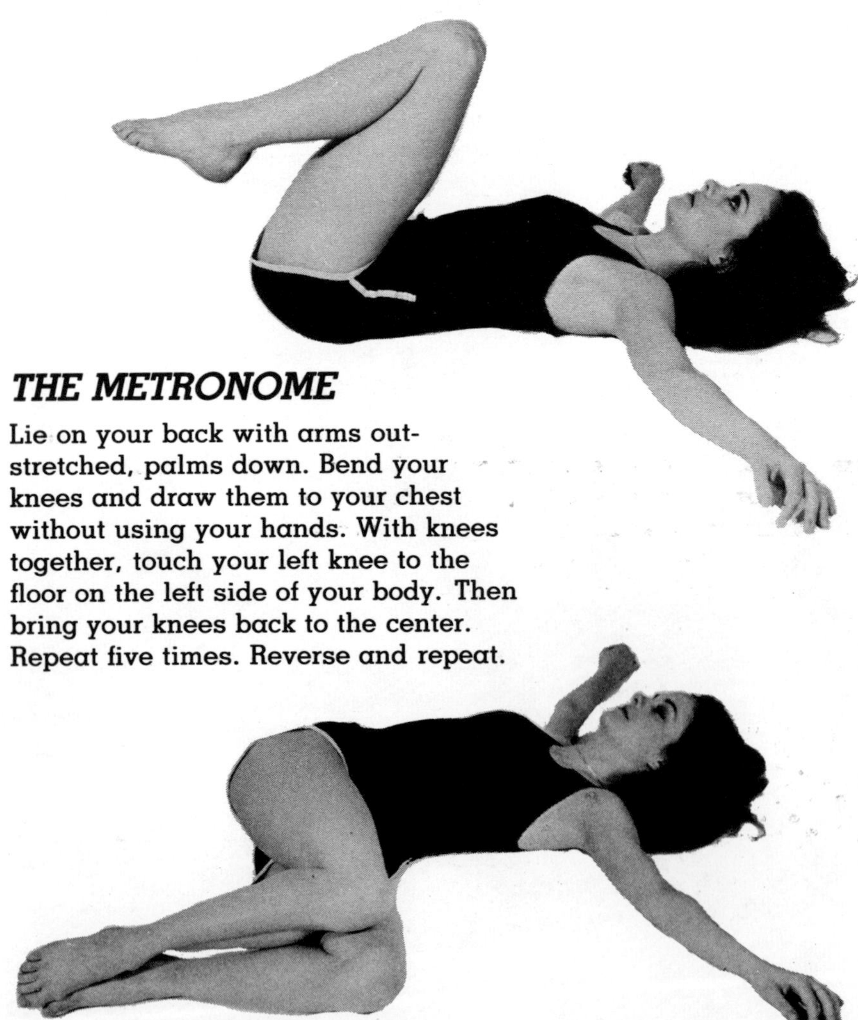

THE METRONOME

Lie on your back with arms outstretched, palms down. Bend your knees and draw them to your chest without using your hands. With knees together, touch your left knee to the floor on the left side of your body. Then bring your knees back to the center. Repeat five times. Reverse and repeat.

THE TRIANGLE

Lie on your right side. Support your body with your right arm only, resting your left hand on your hips. Raise and lower your free left leg five times. Reverse and repeat.

If you have upper back and shoulder problems, try another version of this exercise. Lie on your right side. Then support your upper body at an angle to the floor with both hands, palms down and arms straight. Keep your body rigid as you raise and lower your free leg five times. Reverse and repeat.

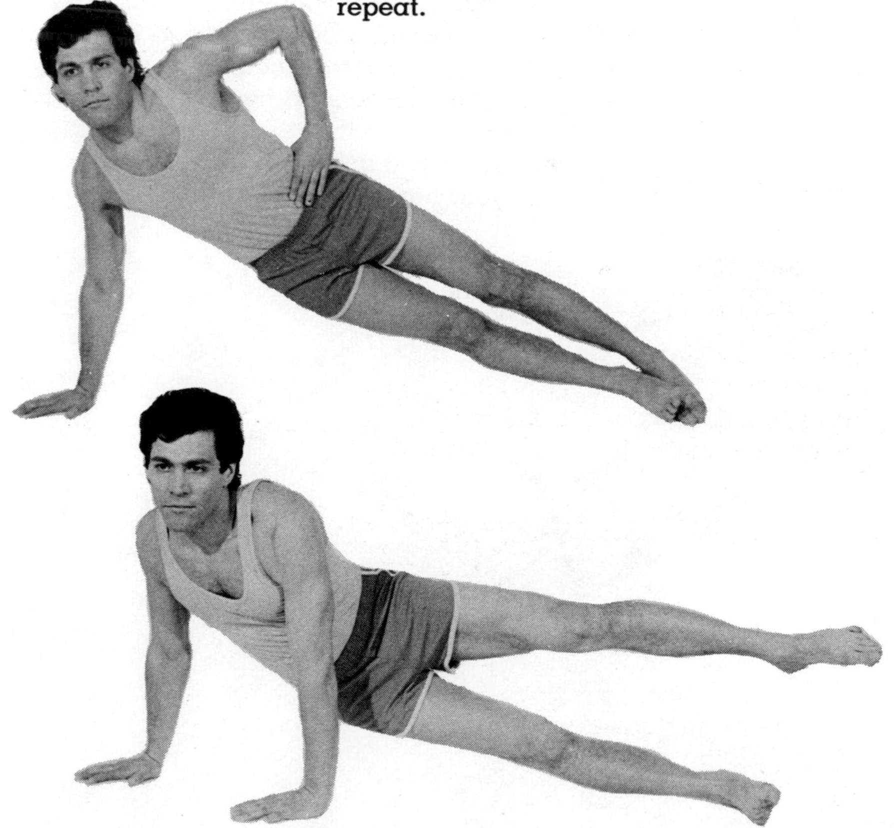

THE CURL WITH TWIST

Lie on your back with fingers interlaced behind your neck or with arms relaxed at your sides. Bend your knees and place the soles of your feet on the floor. Slowly curl your head and trunk off the floor, and then twist your torso slightly to the left without lifting your pelvis. Return to starting position, and lift and twist to the right. Repeat five times. As you do this exercise, do not use your hands to support the lift.

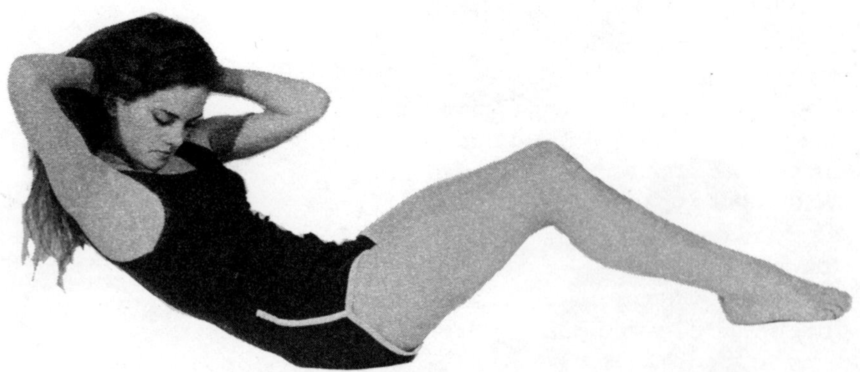

THE SEAL

Lie on your left side with arms in front of you. If necessary, brace your feet under a stable piece of furniture. Slowly raise your head and torso as if doing a half sit-up, and hold the position to the count of five. Do not support the upper body with your hands. Repeat five times. Reverse and repeat.

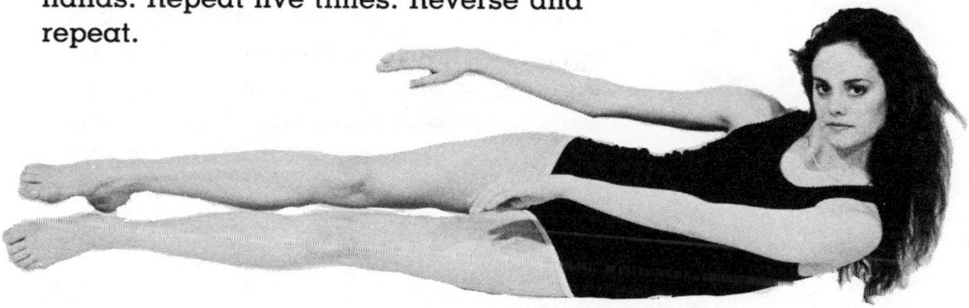

THE ARCH

Sit on the floor with arms raised overhead and spread your legs as far apart as you can without arching your back. With hands touching each other, stretch your torso to the left and try to touch your ankle with both hands. Return to starting position and repeat five times. Reverse and repeat.

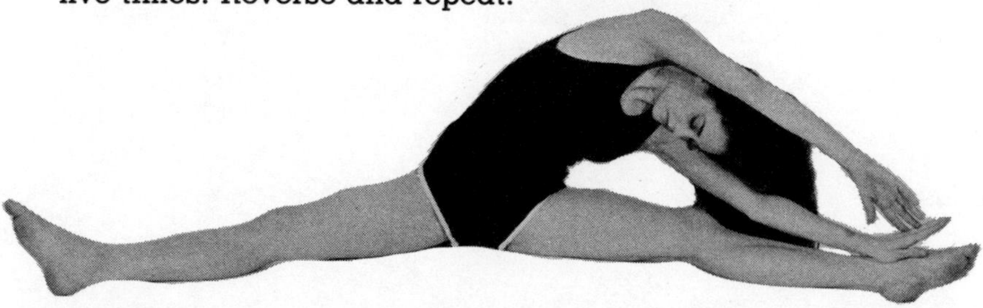

THE SIT-UP WITH TWIST

Lie on your back with fingers interlaced behind your head and knees bent. Gradually raise your torso from the floor with a curling motion, starting with your head and shoulders. As you complete the sit-up, turn your torso so that your right elbow touches your left knee. Repeat five times. Reverse and repeat.

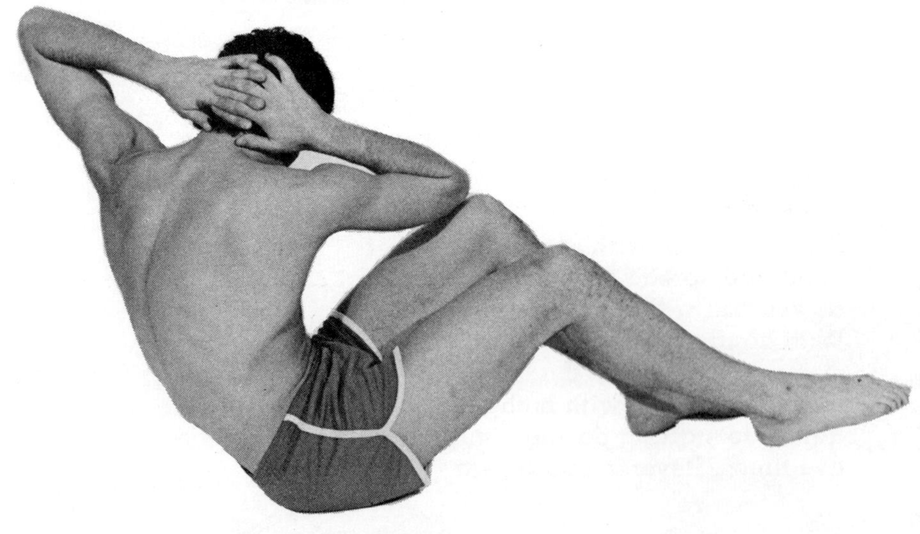

ANYWHERE, ANYTIME EXERCISES

When you have a few free moments during the day, you can put the time to good use by doing some extra exercises. A number of the exercises already described can be done anywhere, anytime; others require only minor adjustments to fit your special circumstances. For example, the first three Warm-ups—the Crescent, the Roundabout, and the Rocker—may be done in an office behind closed doors. Similarly, the Twist from Level 1 and the Rearview Reach from Level 2 can be done as standing exercises, as long as you remember not to sway or tilt your pelvis. Exercising during free moments at the office or elsewhere may even give you an extra burst of energy during a tiring day.

Below you will find some additional torso twists that you can do in your spare time—at home, at the office, or just about anywhere else.

THE TORSO TWISTER

Sitting up straight in your chair, extend both arms in front of you. Twist your torso to the left as far as you can, making sure your pelvis does not move. Then twist to the right. Repeat five times.

THE REACHOVER

Sitting in a chair, extend both arms in front of you. Twist your torso to the left and reach down as if you were picking up an object from the floor. Return to starting position, and then twist and reach to the right. Repeat five times.

THE STRETCH

Stand with feet slightly apart and arms at your sides. Slowly swing your arms to the left and raise them over your head so that you feel the stretch in your left side. Return to starting position, and then raise and stretch to the right. Repeat five times.

THE SHADOW BOXER

Stand with feet slightly apart. Form a circle with your arms in front of you, with your fists clenched. Keeping your pelvis stable, slowly twist your torso as far as you can to the left. Hold the position to the count of five. Then twist to the right and count to five. Repeat five times.

WITH ~ THE ~ HELP ~ OF ~ A ~ PARTNER EXERCISES

The exercises described below should not be attempted alone, but only with the help of a partner. Before actually doing the exercises, it is important for you and your partner to try them out, to run through them without using full strength. This will familiarize you with the stress points and help you to avoid strain.

THE ONE BY ONE

Lie on your back with hands clasped behind your neck. Bend your knees and ask your partner to hold your feet to the floor. Slowly sit up and touch your left elbow to your right knee. Then touch your right elbow to your left knee. Return to starting position. Repeat five times.

THE ROUND THE CLOCK

Lie on your back with arms out at right angles to your body. Keep your feet together with toes pointed down. Raise your legs as high as you can. Your partner grasps the arches of your feet and rotates both your legs in large circles. Make five circles clockwise, then five counterclockwise.

THE ASSISTED SEAL

Lie on your left side with arms in front of you. Your partner grasps your ankles while you slowly raise your torso as far as you can. Repeat five times. Reverse and repeat.

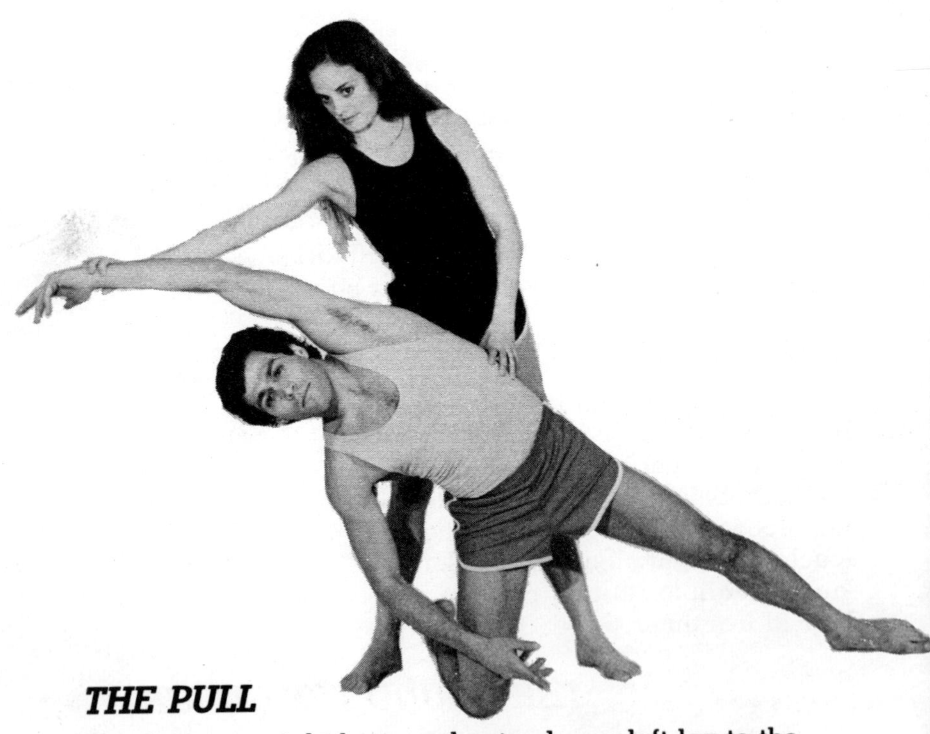

THE PULL

Kneel on your right knee and extend your left leg to the side. Your partner stands behind you. Hold your right hand down in front of you and raise your left hand above your head. The partner grasps your left wrist and pulls the arm downward and to your right. Repeat five times. Reverse arm positions so the partner can help you stretch to the other side. Repeat. Then reverse leg positions and repeat.